END OF LIFE
Tips

BY GABRIELLE ELISE JIMENEZ

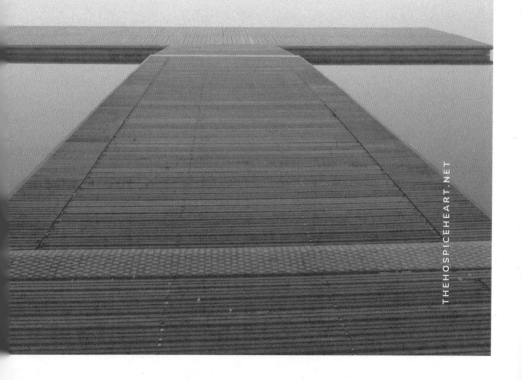

How can we help support someone who is dying?

Meet them where they are, not where you want them to be. We tend to project what we feel and need but their end of life journey is not ours to direct... find out what they need and want, and honor their wishes the very best that you can.

xo
Gabby

ISBN 9798398266580

9 798398 266580

This book is dedicated to my sister Laura and my brother Ben... I will miss you forever.

Forever tucked inside...

by Gabrielle Elise Jimenez

To be gifted someone that loves you
To know that feeling in your heart
To be cared for well, and to feel safe
In life... that is the very best part

Love comes in many forms
And in many different ways
Sometimes it ends way too soon
Sometimes it gets to stay

We never know how long we'll have them
We won't know when they will go
We learn to cherish moments and memories
Life is fragile and precious, that much we know

It is important to remember
That time is an unpredictable gift
And if we try harder not to waste it
Perhaps each moment will be less missed

How can we do this better?
How can we make the best of the time we've got?
I think we absolutely must remember
That time is a gift that cannot be bought

THE HOSPICE HEART

Whether our time with them is long or short
It's not always in our hands
Why they were taken away too soon from us
We will never understand

The hardest thing about loving someone
Is when you have to say goodbye
There is no easy way to do that
You just have to feel, react, and cry

Every minute we are gifted time with them
And all the love they've thrown our way
Is a gift to be held onto tightly
It is ours, never to be given away

So, when it's time to say goodbye
Despite the ache that we will feel
Despite the time that was stolen from us
Despite how many times we cry

Our love for them, and theirs for us will stay forever tucked
inside....

THE HOSPICE HEART

CONTENTS

INTRO

WHEN YOU AREN'T
THERE AT THE LAST
BREATH

BE ON TIME

DON'T TAKE AWAY
THEIR AUTONOMY

WHAT TO DO FOR
SOMEONE WHO'S
GRIEVING

STOPPING FOOD &
WATER

WHY IS IT TAKING SO
LONG?

THE DEATH RATTLE

MEDICATIONS

VISIONS, VOICES AND
VISITORS

CAN THEY HEAR US?

SIGNS THAT SOMEONE
IS NEAR DEATH

SHOULD WE TALK TO
THE KIDS ABOUT DEATH
AND DYING?

LESSONS I LEARNED
ABOUT LIFE THROUGH
DEATH

Intro

I went to nursing school in my late forties specifically to become a hospice nurse. I was caring for a friend of mine who was dying and felt a sense of peace at his bedside, as though it was a chair that had been saved for me until I finally found it. This work is intimate, private, personal, powerful, and lovely. No matter how many last breaths I witness, it always feels like the first. It is such an honor to be present at the bedside for someone who is dying, as well as for those who are saying goodbye.

Each first hello, and last goodbye is a reminder to me that life is fragile, and our time here is unpredictable. I want to be the last kind word someone hears, I want to be the kind of person that makes a difference for others, that inspires them, that reduces their fears, and that reminds them they are not alone. I appreciate life in a way I never have before, and I savor it all... I am pleased when I can start seeing someone early in their diagnosis, because it allows me to get to know them, find out what they want and what their wishes are, and how they want to be cared for as they start to decline. If I am lucky, I meet their families and hear their stories.

Human beings deserve to be cared for well when they are dying; to be heard, to have their thoughts and wishes, and even their fears validated.

I put their needs first. I focus on listening, because I think all human beings deserve to be heard, but also because if we listen, if we lean in and truly hear what people need, we can honor their wishes and care for them well. Each person I meet along my path, teaches me about life, love, kindness, and compassion, all of which are beautiful gems I keep safely tucked inside me.

Meeting them where they are, not where I want them to be, is something I didn't quite understand early on. This was something I learned after realizing their experience is not about me. Meeting someone where they are means putting aside our wishes for them, even when we think they might benefit from them. It means not telling them where they should be in their journey. It begins by listening without judgment, asking questions openly and honestly, and recognizing that they are human, and have their own needs. Our role is simply to honor them.

It is so easy to project what we think someone else needs, and to push our own wants and wishes onto them, but what I think is more respectful, is truly meeting them where they are and honoring them in a beautiful, compassionate way.

I have learned that I don't always have to be there for the last breath, as long as I make the time that I am there valuable for the patient and their family, and that has to be enough for me.

When you work in end of life care you are constantly caught between feeling sad that they are gone, but happy they let go. This is an emotional seesaw we are all continuously learning to find balance on. Do we get attached? Sometimes, yes. I think that is why self-care is that much more important for us to practice. If we stop having an emotional reaction to the end of a life, and the ache people feel when they say goodbye, we should stop doing this work.

When we are at the bedside of someone who is dying, our presence is not always just about them... it is also for those who are preparing to say goodbye. The partner of the person in the bed, has two roles, partner and caregiver, and the lines between them can become blurry. They need our support the minute they take on that second role. And our role (because we have one too), is to reach out and offer them a break, or to make a meal, or pick up groceries. There are so many things we can do for them that won't take up too much time or money. Imagine the difference you can make for them.

The moment you start providing care for another human being, a bond is created, and you become emotionally connected and tied to this person. All the time you spend with them, caring for them, and focusing on their needs, the more you forget your own. YOU need care too and it is essential that you find a way to practice self-care and honor the needs of your own body. And when that time comes when you have to say goodbye to them, this loss will be big and your grief will be real, you cannot do this alone. Please reach out to someone, let them know you need support.

For a long time, I think I felt like if I admitted how hard it was, or how fragile I was feeling, it would mean I was not up to the task of taking on this job, and that perhaps I was too weak to do it. But that is not the case at all, I am fragile, but I am not weak. Weak would be not admitting you have tough days, weak would be not honoring what your body says to you, and weak would be not accepting that you are a human being doing a job that many could never even attempt, which is hard, and sad, and can take its toll... but it is also beautiful and fills my soul, and I wouldn't have it any other way.

At the end of every single day, I ask myself, "what did I do well, what could I have done better, and what did I learn." My reason for this is to keep finding the balance between the blurry lines of end-of-life care, to accept my emotional reaction as the reminder of how truly precious life is, and to always stay focused on what matters most of all, which is that a human being was cared for well, and that is always my goal. Death has taught me to pay closer attention to life. Each last breath that I am present for shocks me because I realize the finality of it, as well as how truly fragile we are as humans, and how blessed we are to have breath, and life.

When you work in this field and experience your own personal losses, you find yourself in between standing so still you are afraid to move and moving forward swiftly, as though it never happened. Neither are healthy.

I have found that facing all my feelings head on, really feeling them, honoring them, and wiping the sticky off them, helps. I call it "sticky," because that is what grief feels like to me... like it's stuck to me, which then becomes stuck to everything I touch. To work in a field where you have to be strong enough to witness difficult moments, and comfort others who are trying to navigate them, you have to take care of yourself and find a self-care routine that can fit nicely into your daily life.

Journaling, blogging, meditation, yoga, running, walking, hiking, cooking, time with family and time with friends... all of this can center and ground you. This work is beautiful, but it cannot be everything you are or do.

I cry easily and often, and there was a time early on that I felt I needed to hold it in. I spoke to one of the hospice doctors about it, and he looked right at me, into my eyes, and he told me to feel whatever I was feeling. He gave me permission to ache for this loss, which was mine too. He told me that in order to be able to do this work well, we have to remember that we are bearing witness to the end of a life. He said that if I should ever stop feeling a sense of sadness witnessing a last goodbye, only then should I be concerned about whether or not I am capable of continuing to do this work. Their experience is not about us and projecting what we think they might need is not helpful. If we meet them where they are, if we truly listen to what they want or need, imagine how that makes them feel. When someone is nearing the end of their life, what I want most of all is for them to feel as though they were cared for well.

THE HOSPICE HEART

One thing it is always important to remember, is that THIS IS NOT ABOUT US. We should not project what we think someone else needs or wants, whether they have a voice or not. It is not for us to say he should or should not be alone when he dies...... I was reminded that it does not matter who someone prays to, kisses, votes for, or how they live ... this is their choice, and it is not for us to judge, insult, ridicule or verbalize any unkind words or energies in their direction.

I am often asked why someone is taking so long to let go, or an even harder question, is why do they have to die? What I have come to realize is that there is no real answer to the why, and there is nothing I can possibly say that would or could change the circumstances of everything that was happening at the time the questions are being asked. Life happens, and then death happens and in between is the space where memories are made, so it reminds us to make the very best of that time. Sometimes we are reminded too late. And when a diagnosis is given, or a life is cut short, the questions we need to ask are, did we live our life well, did we make lasting memories, do the people in our lives know just how loved they are?

For me, at the end of the day, what matters most...... is that all human beings are cared for well when they are dying, despite their choices, their lifestyle or anything else that we might not support, agree with, or understand.

I found this quote by Colin Powell, which I believe says it all...
"Don't just show kindness in passing or to be courteous. Show it in depth, show it with passion, and expect nothing in return. Kindness is not just about being nice; it's about recognizing another human being who deserves care and respect."

If you are providing end-of-life care, you need to know what a difference you will bring to the life of someone who is dying. When you are at the bedside, you offer peace and you offer trust, and in some cases more so than anyone else in their lives. I have witnessed many times the patient sharing things they had never told anyone else, which is usually about their fears and worries about death and dying. Sometimes, patients are afraid to be open with their loved ones, they don't want to add to the pain they are already going through, that is why this role is so important, your role is so important. The advice I give most often, is to listen, not to fix, not to share your thoughts or your opinions, but to hear them and to validate their words. By doing this, you are building trust. And that is a beautiful gift.

When you meet someone who is dying, always remember what this means to them, and what they might be going through. Time suddenly takes on a whole new meaning when yours has been cut short, and it is at this time when you realize you have wasted a lot of time. There might be regret, anger, guilt, sadness, and pain, which can be physical but is often mental or spiritual as well. There is a lot that needs to be worked through before those last breaths are taken, and your role might just be the safe place for them to share.

THE HOSPICE HEART

Being present for someone who is dying, is an honor, one that should never be taken lightly or for granted. When you first meet them, try not to ask them how they are... we know how they are... instead let them know you are pleased to meet them, and that you are there for them in whatever way brings them the most comfort. At the time of that first visit, they may not know what they want or need, they might not know what a gift you are to them, so this is your opportunity to start building that trust. Lean in, and simply say, "it is an honor to meet you." And let the conversation go from there. You are going to make a difference in their life, and I love you for that.

xo
Gabby

When you aren't there at the last breath

Sometimes people will take their last breath after you've left the room to shower, eat, or just take a moment to breathe. You didn't abandon them. I truly believe that some people do not want an audience, or they don't want that to be the last thing you see. They don't take with them who was there at the last breath... they take with them who was there all along.

Be on time

Time takes on a whole new meaning when you are told you have less of it left. Every single minute becomes incredibly precious. Be mindful of that when you tell someone you will be there at a certain time. If you are running late, please call them and let them know. They need to know that they can trust you, that you are reliable, and that you respect their time. It is one of the kindest and most considerate things you can do for them.

Don't take away their autonomy

When someone is given a terminal diagnosis, it can oftentimes feel like you no longer have autonomy, choice, or even a voice. People tend to talk over you and about you, and everyone is making decisions on your behalf. I once heard a husband say to his wife, "please don't speak for me, this is my illness, and I can still talk." One thing I have learned is how important it is to not take away their autonomy, and for as long as they have a voice, listen to it. Ask them what they need or want, hear them, and honor their words. Let them speak for themselves until they can't.

What to do for someone who is grieving

What can you do for someone who is grieving? Check in on them. Often. Listen to them. Be patient with them. Their grief is not about you, and you don't get to tell them how to grieve. And remember that grief never ends, please don't ever tell someone they should get "over it." They will never get over it. Be kind. Grief is hard. Just give them your love.

Stopping food & water

When someone is actively dying, food and water can actually complicate the dying process, making it harder for the body to let go. If your person refuses food or water at the end of their life, respect that. You are not hurting them. The body does not need that when it is trying to let go, in fact, it makes things easier and more physically comfortable for them if they don't eat or drink at the end of their life.

Why is it taking so long?

I have learned that despite the decline of the person, and despite being given medication, (sometimes a lot of medication) the body will wait to let go until it's ready. If their heart is strong... it can sometimes take a while to let go. I think it's important to trust that the body knows what to do, and when it's ready, it will let go. It's not about us ... sometimes we just have to wait.

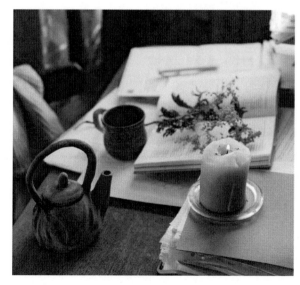

THE HOSPICE HEART

The Death Rattle

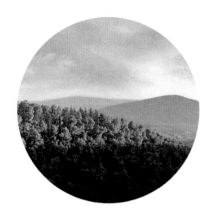

I want to (in my terms) explain the "death rattle", which by the way I think is an awful term, and I wish they would call it something else. I have come to believe that it bothers us more than them. It usually happens at the end of life because our ability to swallow is reduced and we are unable to cough or bring secretions (saliva/phlegm) up or down so it hovers there and will sometimes make a loud vibrating sound, that sounds like rattling, or gurgling.

Please do not rush to get a suction machine or medications like Atropine. First try to reposition them on their side.

Sometimes, that alone can move the secretions just enough to quiet the noise... which again bothers us more than them. Repositioning is oftentimes the remedy.

If the secretions are filling in their mouth, even spilling out, a suction machine is useful, but I want you to imagine what it must be like for the person lying in the bed. The noise is awful, but the suctioning tool is so uncomfortable, and when you are dying, that is the last thing you want happening to you. Try and use mouth swabs to remove the secretions manually first... please... it is so much gentler and far kinder.

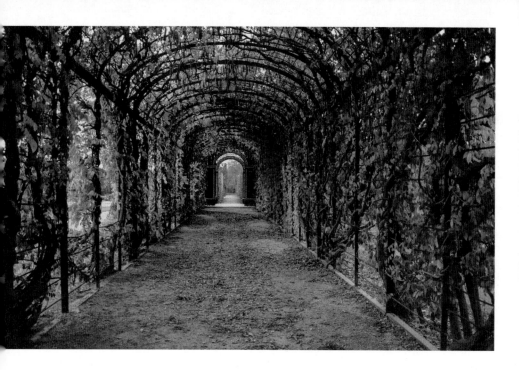

Medications like Atropine are effective, but usually more effective when the secretions are pooling in the mouth, not when they are in the throat or chest. A suction machine is also helpful in that same way. Neither are very helpful when the secretions are down the throat and just hovering there.

My hope in sharing some of these tips/tools is to relieve your fear, and to help you be better prepared for what happens when we die. The death rattle is common at the end of life, and sometimes it does not happen.

To be present for someone when they are dying, means to witness the ways our bodies shut down. It can be messy; it can even be a little scary... but our bodies know what to do and the things we experience are a natural part of the dying process.

Sometimes, I just lean in... I place my hand on their back and rub it gently, whispering... "it's okay, I am right here... I've got you... you are not alone." And that... comforts them. Trust your words, your heart, and your touch... it is amazing what comfort these can bring.

THE HOSPICE HEART

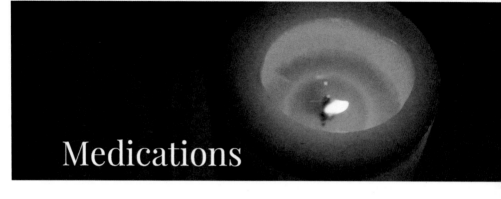

Medications

I will start by saying that I am not a big of fan of using a lot of medication. What I mean, is that it is not usually my first go-to, because I would like to think there are other things we can do first to try and relieve distress, discomfort and/or suffering, such as re-positioning, or providing verbal or tactile stimuli. Even doing things as simple as making sure their clothing is not bunched up against their back, or that their brief is clean and dry can bring comfort and reduce agitation. I like to try these things first.

Medication is important to have on hand and will oftentimes be the difference between pain and peaceful. The medications we commonly use at the end-of-life are Morphine, Lorazepam (Ativan) and Haloperidol (Haldol). These are the ones I am most familiar with, however there are others. I am not afraid of these medications, because I have seen them work effectively and I rely on them.

I am also comfortable with using these medications paired together, I often say "they are good friends, they play nicely together." What this means to me, is that when given together, they can provide more comfort and relief. For instance... if there is pain, it enhances the agitation/anxiety, and if there is agitation/anxiety, it can enhance the pain. If Morphine and Lorazepam are given together, they can oftentimes reduce the symptoms effectively.

While I understand and respect that there is a fear of addiction when using these medications, I do not worry about that at the end of life. If they are struggling in any way, I want to reduce that. I think it is important to acknowledge and address someone who has that fear, but I also want to help them to let it go.

A comment I hear often is the connection between hospice, morphine, and death. I have heard people say that their loved one died when they were given morphine. I have not been in their shoes, I wasn't there when this might have happened, so I can only speak from my own experience and from what I have seen.

Can someone die after taking these medications. Yes. Did you or your doctor or nurse end their life by giving it to them? In my experience I will say no. Sometimes people are struggling, and they are given medication and they die after. My rationale for this is that the medication allowed them to succumb and give into what was already happening to them. Their diagnosis and disease process ended their life, the medication just gave their body permission and the peace to let go. At least that is how I feel...

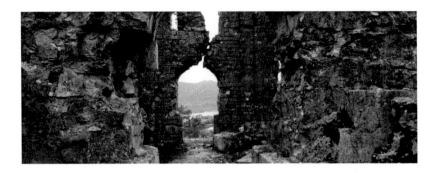

I am also a believer that more is not always better. Our bodies react differently to medication, so we cannot assume that what worked for one person will work for another. This also means that we tolerate doses differently as well; for instance, one person can take Lorazepam and feel relaxed and calm shortly after, but need another dose after thirty minutes, while another person might sleep for an entire day. This cannot be predicted.

I like to wait to see how medication works before immediately giving another dose. I have witnessed someone with pain have their pain increased with more pain medication, so again, more is not always better.

Things to be mindful of when using these medications: Constipation is a common side effect, but the one I usually look for is the dry eyes, the dry mouth, and the reddened and warm cheeks, because this can be uncomfortable to someone who is dying. And this is where you come in... offer a cold compress on the cheeks and eyes, or wetting eye drops for the eyes (check with the doctor first), and even just one drop of water on the tongue is comforting to a dry mouth, but please always be mindful of their swallowing ability. If they are alert and oriented, without swallowing difficulty, I suggest sugar-free candies or watermelon... both comfort a dry mouth.

If you are afraid of the medications being prescribed to someone you love, ask for more information. It is important that you feel confident in what is being given. And if you are the doctor or nurse suggesting a medication, please offer as much information to the family as you can, allowing them to feel confident in what is being suggested. Education is so important, and can many times relieve people of their fear.

Medication is scary, and most people equate it to addiction and death, so I make it a point to do my best to remove these worries from the people who are about to say goodbye to someone they love.

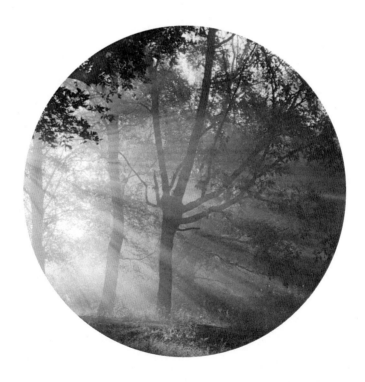

Visions, Voices and Visitors

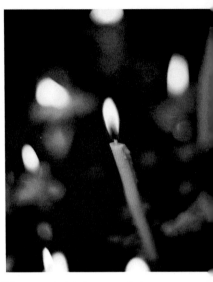

Our role is not to prove someone wrong, but to instead support them if it brings them comfort. Let's place scientific proof, endless data, and opinions of others aside for now...

and imagine that anything is possible. These are just my opinions, what I have witnessed, and how I feel about this topic personally.

I visited a man a few weeks before he died. He told me that his dogs, both of which died years ago and years apart, had started to visit him. His question was, "does this mean I am close to death?"

I first asked about the dogs, their names and whether they were alive at the same time, and how it felt to have them there. He was so pleased they were there, and he told me that they didn't get along well when they were alive and the older one died a few weeks after he got the second, so they didn't have a lot of time together, but now, as they lay on his bed, they were the best of friends. I explained to him that it is my opinion that when someone is near death, they are more open, perhaps spiritually, maybe intuitively, to welcoming the things we cannot see or hear.

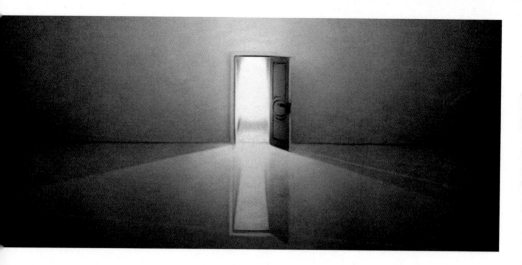

I told him that from my experience it doesn't necessarily determine his timeframe, but that it was my opinion he was close. On the day he died, I was there with him. I asked him if the dogs were there; he patted the bedside (as if to pet them), smiled, and said, "yes." He died about an hour later.

I have witnessed many people seeing friends or family members that have passed away, people they didn't know, one even told me Jerry Garcia played music at her bedside. I have only witnessed one person fearful of what she saw, because it was so startling to her, but soon after, she found comfort with the visits from the stranger. People who can verbalize and are alert and oriented, share their stories with me and I sit, almost child-like at their bedside, eager and excited for every word. Because to me, I see the comfort this brings, but I am also curious, and I want to learn more. In many ways it is a hand stretched out, with someone saying, "I will take your hand and join you on this next part of your journey, so you do not have to do it alone." This works for me.

Some people are no longer verbal, but I can tell they either see or hear something, by the way they gaze (usually at the wall or ceiling), with glazed eyes, and sometimes their arms or hands are stretched out. Family members are worried, they don't understand, most cannot accept it to be true, so they want to talk them out of what they see or hear, convince them they are wrong, or even medicate them out of their "hallucinations." I can appreciate the discomfort the unknown can bring, so I always take time to help those at the bedside feel a little more accepting, and hopefully less fearful.

THE HOSPICE HEART

I have learned that some people can have these visions or hear voices months before they die, some it only happens hours or days before, so this cannot be predicted. Most people do not struggle or feel fear, and for the most part find comfort, safety, and peace. I always encourage families to just listen, and ask questions like, "what do they say?" or "what are they wearing?" If you leave the door open for them to trust you with what they see or hear, they will be more inclined to include you... and trust me, you want to be included.

There can be a darker more uncomfortable aspect to this, which some of you might have witnessed. Terminal delirium is a real thing, hallucinations can happen, and fear is difficult to watch. This is that time when it is so important to talk to the doctors and ask what you can do, and most of the time, medication is key, so my advice is to trust that.

Whether there is a curtain, a veil, or a sparkly silk cloth that comes between us and whatever is waiting for us on the other side, if someone hears a comforting voice or sees an outstretched hand offering safety on their journey, I believe our role is simply to thank them for being there, and feel comforted that someone you love, has a companion to take those next steps with. Instead of questioning or correcting... ask questions and offer them a safe place to talk about the mysteries and magic of the dying process.

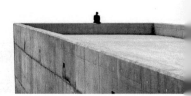

Can they hear us?

When my parents died, a few years a part, I was present for both, but only physically. I didn't know what to say or what to do and no one was there to guide me. Twenty-five years later I am a hospice nurse and the thing I think I do best is provide bedside support to patients and those who are saying goodbye. I always encourage people to say "the things" at the bedside, because I believe if they are said, there will be less regret and possibly even less grief, that they will have to carry the rest of their lives. If I knew then what I know now, I would have sat at my parent's bedsides and at the very least, said goodbye. I have spent all these years wishing I had said so many things.

The first advice I want to give you, is to not wait for the bedside to "say the things." Say them now when you have a chance. Imagine if you didn't have years' worth of held-onto feelings in those last moments, and you could instead simply use that time to say I love you, thank you, and goodbye.

The question that I am asked quite often, is "can they hear me?" I have heard that the hearing ability seems to become heightened at the end of life, but I don't think that is why they hear us.

THE HOSPICE HEART

I think it is our love for one another, our history, our life experiences, our spiritual connection, and the magic and wonder that happens at the end of life when two people have to say goodbye. They hear us, because they feel us and they know we are there and somehow everything we think, feel, and say is handed over to them. I think they need to hear those last words as much as we need to say them, so that is enough for me to be absolutely certain that whatever is said moments before last breaths are taken, are without a doubt heard. Trust that.

While I wish everyone said "the things" way before they find themselves about to say goodbye, I will always encourage people to say whatever they need to before last breaths are taken.

 I imagine their words as a take-away, a beautifully wrapped gift for the person who is dying, to take with them when they go.

Sometimes there is history that is not pleasant, perhaps years of disconnect prior to this bedside moment, which means there are years of unsaid words that there will never be enough time for. But what if you apologized, forgave, or made amends and what comfort that might bring. And if the damage and pain is too deep, what if you simply wished them peace, and said goodbye. This is not a moment to make up for lost time, it is a moment to let go and say goodbye, for you and for them.

I believe that people who are dying need to know a few things; that the people they love will be cared for well, that their name will always be said, and that their legacy will be carried on for many lifetimes. And they need to know, without any doubt, that they were loved. Imagine if we just said those things.

When my brother was in the ICU, I talked to him every single day. He was non-responsive, and he was dying, but I held out hope he would pull through. We had not talked for a long time, so each day I sat at his bedside, I offered and asked for forgiveness for the time we both wasted, I said we would do better if given another chance, I told him I loved him, that I've missed him, and that I was sorry. When he woke up for one day before he died, I asked him if he heard what I said to him. He said, "I'm sorry too."

I believe with every ounce of my being that they hear us, and I want you to believe that too. You may not get a smile, or opened eyes, you may not hear words in response to yours, or feel a tightly squeezed hand... but I can assure you that whatever you say will be received and it will be the last gift you give them.

So, if you find yourself at the bedside of someone who is dying and you love them, let them know, and tell them their life mattered, wish them a safe journey, and say goodbye, because they deserve that. They hear you; I believe this with every ounce of my being.

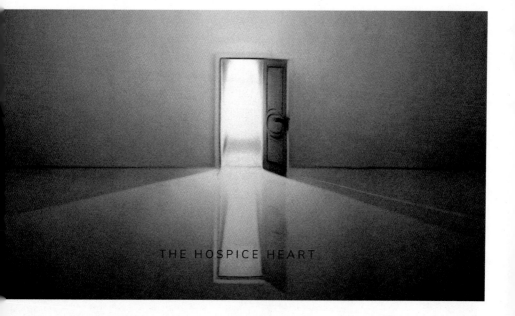

THE HOSPICE HEART

Signs that someone is near death

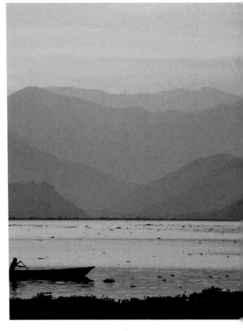

I have witnessed hundreds of last breaths and the one thing I am sure of, is that people do not die the same way. There are many similarities, but I have learned that you shouldn't sit and wait for a specific sign to let you know that someone is about to die. I have heard someone say, "their nailbeds aren't blue, so they aren't close." That person died two hours later.

Nailbeds do turn blue, and the hands and feet can become cool to touch at the end of a life; this can be due to the oxygen level dropping, which is a common sign, but does not always happen. Sometimes their hands and feet are warm up to the last moments before they die. Mottling, purplish or blotchy red/blue coloring on legs or feet, can happen, and is a sign that someone might be close, however it too could never happen.

I have stopped counting on vital signs and will rarely take them, because I find that they can be wrong or misleading and I see the stress it causes families when they stare at the pulse oximeter every twenty minutes.

THE HOSPICE HEART

And I do not understand why people take blood pressure readings when someone is dying, just the thought of that tight squeeze on someone's arm angers me. When someone is dying, the blood pressure will go down, but do we need to squeeze someone's arm tightly while they are in the middle of their dying process to confirm that? I don't think so.

There are many things I look for, that are signs that someone is actively dying, but I never assume one or all will happen. I make sure the families are prepared and know what they can expect to see, because it helps to relieve the fear that can happen at the bedside. Certain signs of death can be scary if no one is prepared.

The dying process and the way the body moves through it, is miraculous. I believe the body knows what to do, and we need to trust that. There are sounds, there are movements, and it can sometimes be frightening, but the sounds and movements are normal and are all a part of the different ways our bodies shut down at the end of life.

I always look in their eyes... they tell me everything. Glazed and glossy tells me they might be close, and when they look as if they are staring beyond you, at something that is a million miles away, that is a sign for me.

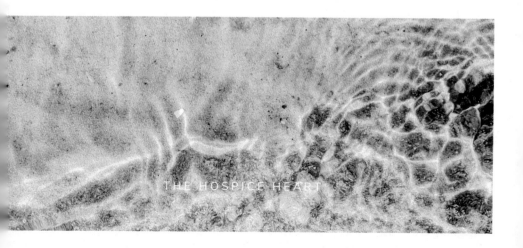
THE HOSPICE HEART

Apnea is a very common sign. This is when they hold their breath, which at first can be 10-15 seconds and a few minutes apart. The first time you witness this, you think to yourself, "this is it," and then they take in a big gasp of breath and go back to their breathing pattern. (I have a three-minute rule and do not assume anything until it has been three minutes.) When they start to hold their breath for longer periods of time, and it begins to happen closer together, that is a sign for me that they are close.

Shallow breathing is a sign that I look for, and mouth breathing, which reminds me of what a fish might do if out of water, is when I know they are very close, and I try to bring the family in.

I always educate the family and let them know about the death rattle, mottling, low oxygen, apnea, body movements, and breathing changes because I want them to be prepared. When it comes down to the last days and hours, the timing is unpredictable... it could happen quickly and quietly and take you by surprise, or they can experience everything that I have mentioned and linger for days. My advice is to not sit and wait for something to happen, but to instead be prepared that it all will. And moments before that last breath is taken, all that really matters is that you are there and that they are cared for well.

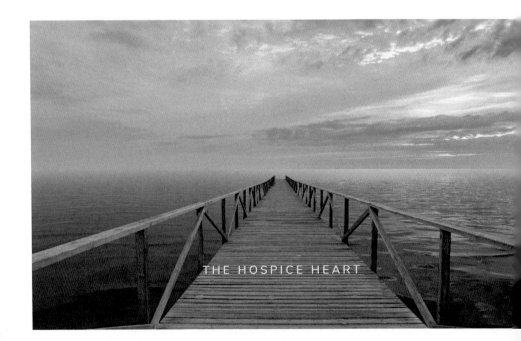

THE HOSPICE HEART

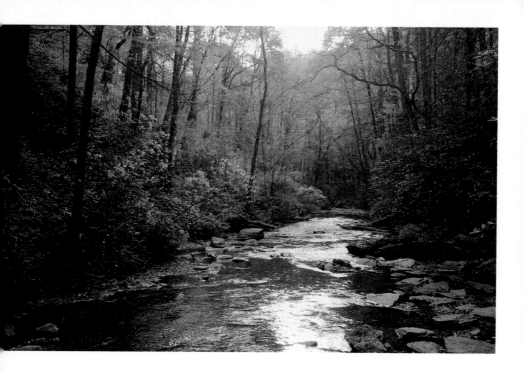

When I start seeing signs that might indicate they are close, I tell the family to assume today is the last day; to sit at the bedside, to say the things, to be fully present and to comfort and support them in whatever ways they might need. And if they are still with us tomorrow, that is a bonus day (more time with them) and you do it all over again. This way they are prepared that it could be hours or days, and less shocked or surprised with the outcome.

There have been times when I have brought the family in, moments before someone takes their last breath, so they can gather to say goodbye; these are beautiful moments. But over time, what I have come to realize is most important, is how prepared someone is for the different ways the human body shuts down. Removing that fear can soften the reaction when someone dies, but remember, no matter how prepared we are, when that last breath is taken, it is as though we had absolutely no idea it was coming.

THE HOSPICE HEART

Should we talk to the kids about death and dying?

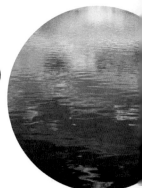

I had my granddaughter over one day and we were coloring when my phone rang. It was the daughter of a patient calling to let me know her mother had died. When I got off the phone I started to cry. My granddaughter asked me what happened, so I told her that someone had died. She asked me why I was crying, and said, "do you love her?" This started the conversation about the work I do, and the reaction I have when someone dies. She equated sadness at death to losing someone (or something) you love. That in itself should tell us that we need to have these conversations with kids.

When we lose a pet, we teach our children to say goodbye, sometimes we even prepare a funeral service of some kind, to honor them. This offers our children the chance to say goodbye, but also to understand and prepare for loss and death. This will never remove the sadness from the loss, but it will prepare them and help them to learn to work through it in a healthy way, helping to remove some of the fear and unknown.

I have a wonderful relationship with my granddaughters, and if I was sick, and if I was dying, I know they would want to be there for me, and at my bedside. Most importantly, I think they would want the chance to say goodbye. Their love for me is real and deep and this would be a difficult loss for them, so I would want to honor that. And them.

If we are not given a chance to say goodbye to someone we love, it adds to the ache we feel and deepens the grief in a way that can many times not be relieved. If children can feel love, they can feel grief, and I believe that it is our responsibility to find a way to prepare them. It must be done carefully though, because we don't want to hit them hard with the realities of death too early on, because that might teach them to hold back from loving fully, anticipating the loss before they even get to experience the love.

Because I am a hospice nurse, and my granddaughters know that I am there for people who are dying, I talk about death and the fact that we will all one day die. I have honest conversations with them about our pets and people we love not living forever, reminding them that moments matter and that we need to appreciate the time we have with them because we never know how long we are gifted them.

I think it is important to let the kids know when someone they love is not doing well, especially if they might die. We should offer them the chance to visit with them, call them, send them drawings or cards, and to say goodbye.

At the very least let them know, so that they can make the decision of whether they want to see them. Give them a choice. I have met too many people who have told me that no one let them know someone they loved was dying, until after they died. Many were not even allowed to go to the funeral, because they were "too young," and they have carried this with them all their lives. Someone else made a really important decision for them and that doesn't feel fair.

My granddaughters at four and six were both capable of hearing difficult truths. I would never assume that this information could be passed on to all four-year-old's though, so please be mindful of each child individually and what you think they can handle.

If we tell our children that someone (or something) they love is sick, and could possibly die, and give them the choice to see them or say goodbye, we are honoring them in a kind and compassionate way and could quite possibly change (for the better) the way they navigate death and dying as they grow up.

Do I think we should tell children when someone is dying? Yes. Children feel love from the moment they are born, and this feeling grows and evolves with them over time, allowing them to build relationships and connections on a level that is beautiful. I believe they should have the chance to visit with and say goodbye to someone (or something) they love.

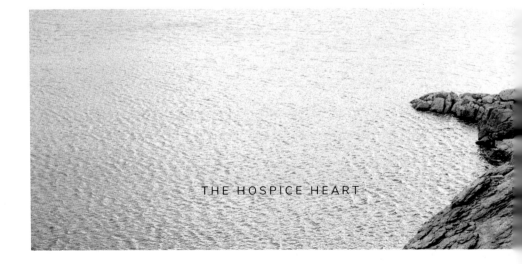

THE HOSPICE HEART

Lessons I learned about life through death

The first death I witnessed was when I was seven or eight years old, and I blocked it out of my memory until I started working as a hospice nurse and wrote my second book, "The Hospice Heart," where I share childhood stories that lighten the path that brought me to do this work. I have seen a lot of death, I have witnessed more "goodbyes" than I can even count, and I have comforted hundreds of people who were about to start their grief walk. I have learned so many lessons about life, through death.

Doing this work has me constantly questioning my own mortality. It makes me more aware of the boxes I want checked off before I go. It has opened my eyes so wide sometimes it burns, to how truly fragile life is, and how so many of us take it all for granted. I have used the phrase, "if I only knew then, what I know now," a billion times. As a hospice nurse, an end-of-life doula, and a conscious dying educator I am waist-high in the river of death and dying and yet, the more I swim here, the less I feel fear, and that comforts me.

I have so many take-aways from this work, so many lessons that I think have helped me to become the kind of person I've always wanted to be, which is someone the people I love would be proud of. Maybe that is my biggest lesson, to live a life where I am my authentic self, and that I leave a legacy behind that my children, their children and even their children will be proud to share.

THE HOSPICE HEART

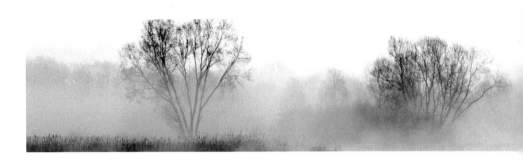

When someone dies, many of us sit at the bedside realizing that we wasted a lot of time. That last breath takes away future conversations, experiences, and memory making so what I am reminded of, is how important it is to do that now while we can.

I have learned that we can't go backwards, we can't call a do-over, we can't take back hurtful or unsaid words, or change situations where we could have done things differently. BUT!!! Death reminds me, that we can do things differently moving forward. It reminds me how truly blessed I am to be alive, to have family and friendships, to do work I am honored to do, to stare at the sky with child-like excitement, to dance like a teenager when my favorite song comes on, and to appreciate every single thing that I have in my life right now, and no longer waste a moment of it or take anything for granted.

From this moment forward, make a difference in this world; for yourself, and for the people who are still standing around you. They matter. YOU matter. Life matters. Let's be kinder to one another, more aware of the struggle's others might be having and extend a hand, or a hug. Let's be the kind of people, that people who love us would be proud of. Nothing is guaranteed, all we can be certain of is right this moment... make it magically delicious!

THE HOSPICE HEART

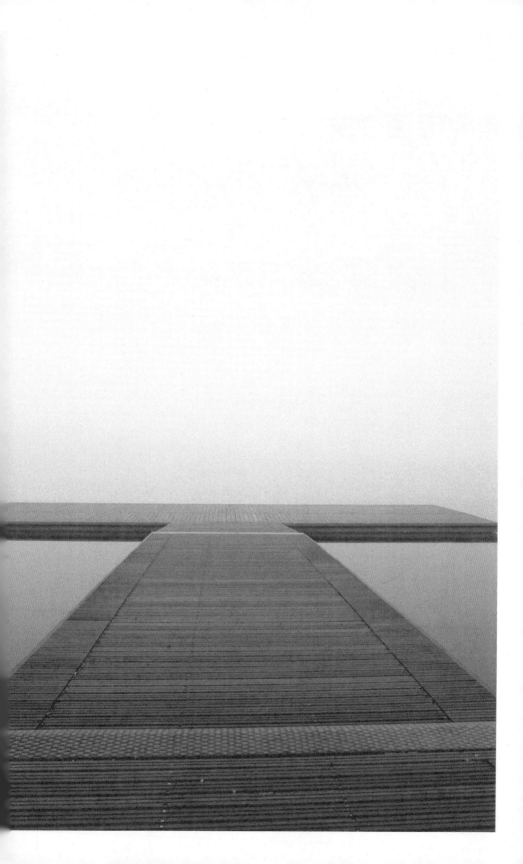

Thank-you

For taking the time to show an interest in end-of-life care, and for helping to improve the way human beings are being cared for when they die.

xo,
Gabby

Contact:

TheHospiceHeart.net

TheHospiceHeart@gmail.com

 @TheHospiceHeart.net

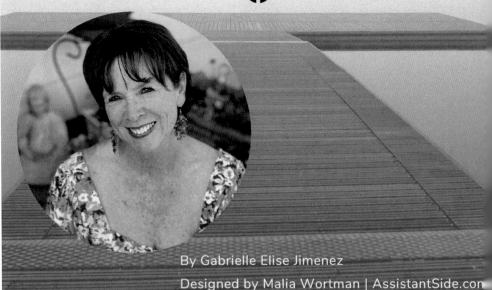

By Gabrielle Elise Jimenez

Designed by Malia Wortman | AssistantSide.com

Made in the USA
Monee, IL
02 August 2023

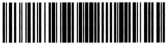

40153651R00026